FAITH
&
FITNESS

Tony B. Milton

Faith & Fitness © 2020 by Tony Milton. All Rights Reserved.

All rights reserved. No part of this book may be reproduced in any form or by any electronic or mechanical means including information storage and retrieval systems, without permission in writing from the author. The only exception is by a reviewer, who may quote short excerpts in a review.

Scripture quotations taken from the Amplified® Bible (AMP), Copyright © 2015 by The Lockman Foundation
Used by permission. www.Lockman.org

The Holy Bible, New International Version®, NIV® Copyright © 1973, 1978, 1984, 2011 by Biblica, Inc.® Used by permission.
All rights reserved worldwide.

Cover designed by J. Dortch Graphic Designs
Printed in the United States of America
First Printing: December 2020
The Scribe Tribe Publishing Group

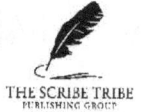

ISBN-978-1-7358251-9-9 (print)
IBSN-978-1-7362882-1-4 (electronic)

ACKNOWLEDGEMENTS

I would like to thank all the people who played a part in the inspiration and completion of this book.

To my Lord: I would like to thank my Lord and savior Jesus Christ for being the center of all things good and true!

To my parents: I would like to thank you for always allowing me to be able to grow in my potential and encouraging me to be all that God has called me to be. I love you!

To my friends and family: I want to thank you all for befriending me and loving in all phases of my life. Love you guys!

CONTENTS

Acknowledgements 1
Introduction 3
Day One 8
Day Two 14
Day Three.. 21
Day Four 28
Day Five 35
Day Six 42
Day Seven 49
ABOUT THE AUTHOR 55

INTRODUCTION

In the beginning God created the heavens and the earth. After some time, He saw that it was good, and He rested. This closure was given after all that He desired for the creation of existence was conquered. God had a plan for us since the beginning of time and that plan was to make sure that we became the best versions of ourselves He created for us. This is not a book helping you to get right and tight within 60 seconds, nor is it going to be anything other than a very honest look at our quest for better and more. We are all on a journey to find better and to become better but to do so, we must look at what it takes to get there. It is totally important, but unfortunately uncommon, to desire greater for yourself; this book hopefully will change that. My desire for people is that we can develop the courage to work toward having more. From our birth, we were shaped and molded to become responses to what happens to and around us. This only leads me to believe that who we are might not be who we were created to be. There comes a time in every individual's life where we question our lives and our decisions thus far. At this point things like depression try to creep in and make us regret and resent our life story, when truly who you are to become is being built of the very thing you hate about your history. This book will express areas of life we, in most cases, have casually looked past. In this book, I attempt to bring clarity to the very small details that have created noticeably big stumbling blocks in our process of growth. Growth is a process and it takes information to be able to navigate through that process. I genuinely believe that the word of God has given us extremely helpful outlooks and insight as to how to maneuver the path of our life story. The Bible says in John 1:1: **"In the beginning was the Word, and the Word was with God, and the Word was God."** This only brings me to believe that the word of God is the origin of all existence, thus ultimately becoming the answer to all the problems existence might have to offer. In the next seven days, my goal is to be able to unlock the desire in you to obtain greater. To get you to taste test what applying your

God-given greatness can potentially get you. Seeing the possibilities only becomes effective when you take the step to apply energy toward what it is you visualize. The sky is literally the limit for you and it's truly up to you to rewrite your own story. We can achieve growth by the adjustments we make day by day and week by week. We learn in life that this process to more is a marathon not a sprint but taking the small steps to change will create big differences. Every day we have 24 hours to make our greatest attempts to create another reality for our lives and taking advantage of those hours is what gives you your God gifted purpose. By way of the death of Jesus, we are given the right to be as great as we desire to be. So, in the next seven days I hope you allow yourself to push personal limits shattering your own stereotypes in your thinking, your spirit, your body, and emotions. This is our gift of a new birth and it's where everything changes for the better!

DAY ONE

Decisions, Decisions...

"I keep my eyes on the Lord. With him at my right hand, I will not be shaken." Psalm 16:8 NIV

Life is all about decisions and unfortunately, most times the most important and beneficial decisions are the hardest to make, taking the longest to set in. The Bible says to *set the Lord before you*, which means to purposefully place a thing in front of yourself. In order to begin to work towards the better us that you dream and envision for yourself, everyday it is imperative that you allow the Father who controls heaven and earth to go into your day before you even get to it. New habits and lifestyles are uncharted territory. So, most of the obstacles that come, naturally you've never seen or dealt with before. This morning the prayer is to make sure that we allow God to know that before we go into our day that He goes before us to clear the path of obstacles and traps the devil has set before us. Newness can seem painful and most definitely is not easy, but on the contrary will be the most beneficial struggle of your life.

The Lord is at my right hand. The best place you want God to be is at your side. So not only will He go before you to clear your path, but He will also come back to walk by your side along the way. In the time of trouble, you need the savior to be by your side to show you how to go around, jump over and fight through the mental and physical battles the day is going to present. Today, in pursuit of establishing a renewed life and building a stronger relationship with the Savior, we make sure that we place Him as the focal point of our day by deciding on purpose to pursue the new He has for us. A new process to *not be shaken* is to develop the mindset of fearlessness, not being controlled by the powers of intimidation which seek to stagnate your pursuit of better. We make a definite decision to not be shaken by the fears of new or by hardship in a foreign place and stage in our life. Being shaken by the spirit of fear only prolongs the process of establishing life habits both spiritually and physically for the growth your next season needs. So, this being our first day into our new journey, we seek guidance from God this morning to go before us, stand beside us and build up our faith to shun the spirit of fear.

SCHEDULE OF THE DAY

MORNING PRAYER

Father, we thank You for this day and repent for all we have done to go against Your plan for our lives. We ask that You go before us this morning and prepare the path that You have for us to go. As we transition into this new level of disciplined life we have chosen, help us to remain resolute with our decision to grow. We give You our lives to use and groom. In Jesus' Name we pray, Amen!

MEDITATIONAL SCRIPTURE

"The Lord himself goes before you and will be with you; he will never leave you nor

forsake you. Do not be afraid; do not be discouraged." Deuteronomy 31:8 NIV

WORKOUT OF THE DAY

- CARDIO: 20 minutes Walking on treadmill or elliptical
- LEGS: 4 sets of 15 Bodyweight Squats (3-second pause between each rep)
- ARMS: 4 sets of 12 Bicep Curls (3-second pause between each rep and back against the wall to prevent swaying)
- SHOULDER: 4 sets of 10 Alternating Lateral to Front Raises (slightly bend the knees for balance)
- ABS: 4 sets of 7 Weightless Russian Twists (left to right is one rep)

DAY TWO

He Knows Me

The word of the Lord came to me saying, "Before I formed you in the womb I knew you, before you were born I set you apart; I appointed you a prophet to the nations." Jeremiah 1:4-5 NIV

Being born on this planet, we have all been given a destiny and a promise of purpose. God who controls all things has given us all a predestined plan in life. In the beginning of time, the God who holds the keys to heaven and earth and is mentioned in many cases as the beginning and the end, formed you and shaped you to be a visual demonstration of His power and glory. This holds true both physically (in your look and lifestyle) and spiritually (your ability to demonstrate His personality through yours). In order for you to be what you have been formed and shaped to become, it is very important you become resolute in the fact that change is never easy and in the beginning of anything you might be completely terrible. It is a form of pride that causes one to believe that everything we put our hands to accomplish we will always be the best at, even if in the first stages of doing it. This harsh reality comes if you have a fear of not being the best or instantly excelling, which only exposes your fear of people's opinions. A fearful lack of being accepted by peers has begun to creep into your life. The mental resolution demands that you come to a permanent place in your mind that declares your decision to change how you walk, how you talk, your relationships with God and people.

You were born to be great and before the earth came into existence He knew and planned your greatness. Your mentality (once resolute with destiny and the life it requires) becomes one of purpose-driven persistence. You wake up in the morning with the Lord's purpose for the day on your lips and in your mind because you know that before you were born your destiny to national and legendary greatness was already established. God loves for us to awaken in the morning declaring and decreeing His will and purpose for our lives. We must also understand and remember that words have power. Our words create volume, pace, and grants either victory or defeat depending upon what words we use to shape the day. God being Lord over our past, present, and the future gives us true insight into getting the victory over today for the rest of our lives. So, this morning we awaken knowing that our lives have already been shaped and the path to success is already made, so the only thing you must do is walk in it. Brush your teeth in success, eat breakfast in success, hit the gym in success, and clock into work in success because it is so.

SCHEDULE OF THE DAY

MORNING PRAYER

Jesus of Nazareth, we come before You today thanking You for waking us up this morning by Your mighty hand. We repent for not acknowledging You as God and Lord over all things great and small. So, we now live in the knowing of our destiny already being made plain in our future. We will become, through the resolving of our minds, bodies, and souls, everything that You have called us to become. We look forward to our futures in You, Lord, and greatness that will come as a result. Our hearts yearn to please You and we are willing to live out the changes to do so. In Jesus' Name we pray, Amen!

MEDITATIONAL SCRIPTURE

"For I know the plans that I have for you, declares the Lord, plans to prosper you and not to harm you, plans to give you hope and a future." Jeremiah 29:11 NIV

WORKOUT OF THE DAY

- CARDIO: 30 minutes on the Stairmaster or treadmill
- CHEST: 4 sets of 11 Pushups (3-second pause between each rep. If unable to do full pushups, you can allow knees to touch the floor)

- LEGS: 4 sets of 13 Bodyweight Lunges (Left and Right leg equals one rep)
- BACK: 4 sets of 12 Seated Lateral Cable Pull Downs (4-second pause between each rep)
- ABS: 4 sets 35-second planks.
- STRETCH: 30 minutes (15 minutes upper body and 15 minutes lower body

DAY THREE

Early Rising

"In the morning, Lord, you hear my voice; in the morning I lay my requests before you and wait expectantly." Psalm 5:3 NIV

We often hear phrases like "the early bird gets the worm" and most times when we hear things repeatedly it tends to lose its significance in our hearts and minds. Though very commonly stated it is true and beneficial to any change and increase in levels of discipline and work ethic. When changing our life patterns in terms of our devotional habits, our emotions, and patterns involving our physical health, we only give ourselves a greater head start on successful changes if we allow our morning to be carefully planned. Morning prayers with declarations to devote our days in our prayer time with God allows Him to have free rein over our 24 hours. The best time to get ahead of the traps the devil might have planned for today is in the morning. Eagerly watching, praying, and stewarding over the day keeps the victory for the day in our corner.

One of the biggest benefits to serving a God who lives and breathes is the fact that He can also hear. Yes! He certainly hears us, in our ups He hears, in our downs He hears, when we cry, He hears and in our rejoicing

He hears. When you call, His heart's desire is to hear the voices of His people, but when you get His ear it is important to be certain in what you send into the heavens. Understanding the influence that the spirit has on the earth is enormously powerful for one to learn the power of binding and loosing demonic and angelic spirits over the day. The hearing of the ears of God allows us access to the throne of grace where our healing and protection in our daily journeys come from. The attention of God's ears are an advantage most of us unfortunately have not learned to capitalize on. Before you can allow the opinions, doubts, and weariness of the day to set in, take full advantage of the privilege to speak to Him.

It's the work done early that predicts great possibility to victory. Good prayer and meditated devotion gives us a pattern of victorious thinking in what we choose to eat, the effort we put into the betterment of our physical selves (fitness and health), and how diligent and humble we are toward our jobs and lives surrounded by them. The Bible constantly teaches foundations and the best way to see your mornings is as the foundation of the day. Truthfully, whatever we choose to make our foundation (whether positive of negative) will manifest the outcome of a victorious or defeated day. We have been blessed with another day, which is another chance to be all that we are born to be, so let us build our day on making sure God hears our voice and that we eagerly watch, stewarding the day to see our prayers and decrees through.

SCHEDULE OF THE DAY

MORNING PRAYER

O Lord, we love You this morning for being Lord over our lives and we honor You for being everything we could never be for ourselves. We repent for not being aggressive in our attempts to love You more and make Your purpose true and first in our lives. We acknowledge that You hear us, and we acknowledge that You see us, so we want to use Your ears to declare and decree the wonderful spirit of health and healing over our lives and our days. We arise early this morning to post You, Lord, as the beginning and the end of this day and declare that is it Your glory will be fulfilled in our day. Peace and Prosperity will be our portion. In Jesus' Name we pray, Amen!

MEDITATIONAL SCRIPTURE

"The LORD is far from the wicked (and distances Himself from them), But He hears the prayers of the (consistently) righteous (that is, those with spiritual integrity and moral courage)." Proverbs 15:29 AMP

WORKOUT OF THE DAY

- CARDIO: 30 Minutes Walking on Treadmill with Incline
- ARMS: 4 sets of 15 Triceps Cable Pull-Downs (3-second pause between each set)
- LEGS: 4 sets of Straight Leg Deadlifts (3-second pause and please see

instructions on how to properly perform before attempting)
- ABS: 4 sets of 12 Seated Jack-Knives/ Scissor (3 second pause in between each rep)

DAY FOUR

I've Got the Victory!

"But thanks be to God, who always leads us as captives in Christ's triumphal procession and uses us to spread the aroma of the knowledge of him everywhere."
2 Corinthians 2:14 NIV

By day four you've made it past the place of deciding and becoming resolute with your choice to make some changes for increase in your life. Today, we are now in a place where we need

God's strength to help us through the fight. Because consistent prayer/devotion (in some cases) and physical exercise may be a new addition to your life, fatigue and a bit of soreness will begin to set in. Unfortunately, when the body begins to feel fatigue and weariness it tends to want to question if we actually have the will power to even continue the path to better, questioning if it's worth it. The truth is you don't by yourself have the will power to sustain the mental or physical energy at the level to see persistent change. It is going to take something greater than you to carry you into place of triumphal victory. What we fail to realize is that He becomes our strength and gives us the victory to spread the knowledge of where true victory and greatness comes from. Jesus leads us through the triumph of pain and fear in a processional. He parades the victory He has graciously given us through His death and resurrection. Our lives are supposed to be living, breathing, walking, and talking representations of the glory of God. Our love to others represents His love to us, the peace in our lives represents His peace toward earth, our ability to bless others represents His ability to bless us, and our success in our living represents His success in governing the earth.

The knowledge of who Jesus is can be compared to a "fragrance" in that it is the sweetest, most wonderful thing you could ever encounter. What better to spread throughout the earth than something that is sweet, wonderful, joyful, peaceful, victorious, takes away fear, pain and ultimately brings light to the earth? In the 24 hours that God blesses us to have each day, it will take God and God alone to give you the strength you need to be the greatness you were born to be. There is a version of ourselves we have never seen that change and progress is trying to push us to. We surely must know that stepping beyond the "us" we've always known will take something beyond ourselves to accomplish. The triumph gives us hope that we will get the victory in the many battles to come. The victory over today will give us faith that the same God that gave us this victory will surely give us the next. Remembering why He gives the triumphal procession is the most important factor to understanding purpose. It's the spreading of the knowledge of Jesus Christ that makes Him give us the victory before the fight even starts; it's all worth the investment. So, on this day we will awaken understanding that the triumphal procession is our parade of the victory in Jesus Christ.

SCHEDULE FOR THE DAY

MORNING PRAYER

Lord of heaven and all things under the heavens, we thank You for this day and honor Your presence in our lives as our provider and as the author and the finisher of our faith. You are King of kings and Lord of lords and we repent for not recognizing You as the Lord you are. We promise to live our lives in the certainty of the triumphant procession already being in our favor and that our lives were given to us solely to spread the knowledge of who You are. We decree our lives to be dedicated to the Lord for Your purpose. We live in the success and greatness of Jesus Christ for the advancement of His kingdom and it will be so! In Jesus' Name we pray, Amen!

MEDITATIONAL SCRIPTURE

"But you are a chosen people, a royal priesthood, a holy nation, God's special possession, that you may declare the praises of him who called you out of darkness into his wonderful light." 1 Peter 2:9 NIV

WORKOUT OF THE DAY

- CARDIO: 30 minutes on the Elliptical (2 minutes accelerated & 2 minutes decelerated)

- CHEST: 4 sets of 12 Dumbbell Flyes (3-second pause between each rep)
- CHEST: 4 sets of 12 Dumbbell Bench Press (3-second pause between each rep)
- LEGS: 4 sets of 11 Dumbbell Step-ups (use bench or any elevated platform; left and right leg is one rep)
- ABS: 4 sets of 10 Leg Raises (lie on your back and lift your legs all the way up with both legs pointed straight; count 5 seconds from bottom to top between each rep)
- STRETCH: 30 minutes (15 minutes upper body and 15 minutes lower body)

DAY FIVE

Humble Pie

"For those who exalt themselves will be humbled, and those who humble themselves will be exalted." Matthew 23:12 NIV

God in His infinite wisdom grants us the blessing of receiving victories we never worked for and truly never deserved. The only downside to serving a God who spoils you with so much favor and liberty is that we occasionally tend to become drunk in the ideas of our hard work or our ability to problem solve. We mistake our skillset as being the reason for the successful victories we have throughout our lives. This becomes more and more of a problematic mindset as time goes on because what begins to rise in us is a sense of self sustainability which then manifests a spirit of pride. Pride is not always a loud and rambunctious attitude but can sometimes be a small notion of deserving certain levels of respect and placement because of one's hard work. The harsh reality is no matter how hard we work; it is the heavenly Father who gives us the ability to work as hard as we do and the favor to allow our hard work to count for something. We have nothing and can accomplish nothing without the Father, and we must always allow that to be the mindset that leads our lives. Victory is only victory when given by the one who holds the keys to everything victorious. It is a human trait to lose sight of where our help comes from. So, to always keep things in perspective just begin to remind yourself that it is God who gives light to the earth, who breathed life into man, who even allows the blood to flow through your veins. The truth is without any of these things being in place we have no way to display the hard work.

Humbleness is a gift and something that it takes a lifetime and a half to perfect but with God, whether voluntarily or involuntarily, He helps us discover ways to keep ourselves humble. It is in humbleness we find our ability to increase. "God refuses the proud" so most definitely He will accept and grant favor to those who remember that all we are and have comes from above and not ourselves. Permanent and persistent change will only cement itself in our lives through the consistent idea that we are not superheroes that can guarantee successful victories in every situation. Admitting our weakness in our humanity only frees us of the responsibility of being our own lord and savior. His job is to keep our best interest in mind, and it's only right that we as His children allow Him to do so. God's job as our father is to correct us when we as humans allow ourselves to become intoxicated by the effortless victories we're blessed to be gifted with. Truthfully, if God was to ever take His hands off us and pull back the favor that He has so richly blessed us with, then we would truly see how unworthy and incompetent we are. Freeing yourself of the burden of having to keep yourself means knowing that it is in Him that we are given life. Humbling yourself is the way to get every blessing God has for us and on this day, we remove ourselves and allow Him to be the great God He is!

SCHEDULE FOR THE DAY

MORNING PRAYER

Father, we pray that You hear our cry for more of You. Lord, we depend totally on Your ability to be God in our lives. We repent for all the things we have done to violate and disrespect Your commandments for the lives of Your children. We repent for allowing the battles You win on our behalf to go to our heads and for forgetting that it is You who keeps us and not we ourselves. We say within our hearts that we will live for the purpose of Your glory in spreading the knowledge of who You are. We will forever acknowledge You for every success, every victory, and ounce of progress You promote in our lives. It is for the advancement of the kingdom that You shine Your light on us and we will forever live in that truth. We bind and break every spirit of pride and forgetfulness that is trying to creep itself in our lives to stagnate our exaltation. We will humble ourselves and allow You to exalt and expand who we are. In Jesus' Name we pray, Amen!

MEDITATIONAL SCRIPTURE

"When pride comes, then comes disgrace, but with humility comes wisdom." Proverbs 11:2 NIV

WORKOUT OF THE DAY

- CARDIO: 30 minutes of Jump Rope (beginners start with a goal of 15 straight jumps)
- ARMS: 4 sets of 15 Skull Crushers (triceps workout)
- LEGS: 4 sets of 10 Bodyweight wide/regular/pencil Squats (10 of each alternating)
- CALVES: 4 sets of 20 Calf Raises (weightless or with weight)

DAY SIX

Internal Warfare

"For though we live in the world, we do not wage war as the world does. The weapons we fight with are not the weapons of the world. On the contrary, they have divine power to demolish strongholds."
2 Corinthians 10:3-4 NIV

Throughout this process of change within the book we have discussed over and over the mental resolutions of our desire for change for our betterment. To protect our decision to change, we war within ourselves internally against opposing spirits that come against the mind (where all decisions are made) and emotions (in what energy all decisions are carried out). We are most definitely human beings that are made up of skin cells and a nervous system. Nevertheless, there is a deeper volume that helps support the reality of our lives and that is our soul. Our cell-filled bodies work and function in a natural sense, but our soul functions in a world that cannot be seen-- the spirit. So, when we are dealing with the warring of our minds and emotions, thoughts and feelings are not things you can see with a magnifying glass. It takes warfare in the unseen to deal with the problems of the unseen. Constant pushing and stretching to provoke progress will always create a place of resistance from ourselves and demonic elements that try to kill our faith in the power that God has richly given us. Fear, Shame and Doubt are some of the internal wars that begin in places of wanting and desiring more. Fear can come in two ways; one is fearing you don't have what it takes to become the success you desire in life. Two is the fear that once you do become successful questioning if you have what it takes to sustain that level of success. Both ideals of fear are brought to your mind by an inaccurate understanding of the role you play in your own success. The Bible specifically says, "I Am the one who takes down one and puts up another." It is not we ourselves that grant promotion or increase, but it is the Lord. You being good enough to arrive and excellent enough to stay is not your job; your only job is to be available.

Satan's plan for creating senses of fear, doubt and weariness is to cloud our minds with so much doubt in God's ability that our minds, bodies, and souls are no longer available for His use. In order for God to use our lives for His glory, He needs our minds to think like His, our souls to feel like His and our bodies to look like His (in the sense of what people see when they look at us).

The Father gives us tools like the word of God, prayer and fasting as ways to build up authority in the world of the unseen. The ability to learn, understand and discipline yourself in the ideals of God and His word arms us with weaponry needed to battle within our minds and souls. The decreeing of blessings and denouncing of darkness is key in sustaining the progress of change. So, this morning we awaken at war to preserve and protect our right to progress and not be hindered or stagnated by the devil's attempts to create **F**alse **E**ntities that **A**ppear **R**eal!

SCHEDULE FOR THE DAY

MORNING PRAYER

Dear Father, we come to You today to say thank You for Your grace and mercy. We thank You for keeping us and believing in us and our future even when we didn't believe in ourselves. We war in our minds to pursue change fighting the thoughts and ideas of weariness, weakness, fear, and doubt. The battle against spirits and principalities are never easy but it is You that is our victory. We repent for allowing our faith in You to be shaken, being weak minded and easily sifted in our beliefs in who You said You are to us. We love You and today we claim our mental and spiritual victories over today. In Jesus' Name, Amen!

MEDITATIONAL SCRIPTURE

"Submit yourselves, then, to God. Resist the devil, and he will flee from you." James 4:7 NIV

WORKOUT OF THE DAY

- CARDIO: 30 Minutes on the Treadmill (walk 1 minute and run 1 minute)

- ARMS: 4 Sets of 15 Bicep Curls (5 from bottom to halfway, 5 halfway to top, 5 all the way)
- LEGS: 4 Sets of 12 Singles Leg Squats
- BACK: 4 Sets of 12 Seated Rows/Cross Body Extension
- ABS: 4 Sets of 12 Decline Sit-ups

DAY SEVEN

The Gift of Rest

**In peace, I will lie down and sleep, for you alone, Lord, make me dwell in safety.
Psalm 4:8 NIV**

Aaaaahhhhhh!! Take a deep breath and relax! You've made it through the first week that will give birth to some of the most productive times of your life. The beginning of a thing is most times the hardest part of a sufficient and sustainable change. There is a sense of pride one should have in certain levels of accomplishment, especially when it involves embarking on something you've never encountered before. God loves to see our reach to become better and our fight against our nature to stay comfortable and stagnate. He loves it when we take the power He has already given us in this earth and utilize it to become the greatest and brightest versions of ourselves within His purpose for our lives. God being Alpha and Omega and the Beginning and the End has already seen the overcoming outcome into the very interesting journey our lives entail. God created the earth in 6 days and on the 7th day he rested; He rested to observe His work and marvel at how great a work He produced. Sometimes it is good for us to sit back and give God thanks, glory, and honor for the wonderful works He has done through us, and also pat ourselves on the back for being available enough to be used in such a beautiful way.

Growth and change are both beautiful and ugly in the same sentence in that the finishing product of change is always glorious but the process getting there can sometimes be brutal. There is a badge and medal of honor one gets when deciding to stick it out through the constant wars of change. So, congratulations because these past 7 days have qualified you for the rewards of warriors. It's not easy changing everything you knew to be a normal place in your life and truthfully there is no quick fix. One of the worst things a person could ever do is trick themselves into putting a concrete limit of time on changes in life. It can be incredibly stressful trying to fulfill a commitment of a deadline when the very thing you're trying to achieve you've never done before. Unfortunately, if we have embarked on this journey before but did not see it all the way through, we can sometimes approach things with the mindset of, "I already know what I'm doing." When in fact you're only educated up until the point that you've completed. Anything past that point is unknown territory.

Day 7 is the day you meditate on how far you've come and what it took to get thus far. Thank God for giving you the grace to survive the ups and downs of this season. Lastly, rest well and mentally prepare yourself for the challenges ahead. It's not going to be easy but to be honest, the idea of becoming the greatest you you've ever seen should sound a little exciting. You've done wonderful; now let's give these goals and dreams a run for their money!

SCHEDULE FOR THE DAY

Morning Prayer

Father, I thank You for being faithful, loving, kind, and peaceful. You are everything we could never be to ourselves. You are the leader and guider of our lives and we give our days to You. You are glorious and Your ways are perfect before our eyes. We thank You for helping us to become brave enough to embark on a journey that will change our lives and the way we live it forever. It was not easy and at times we wanted to quit, but it is You who gives us strength to persevere through trials and obstacles. You have already redeemed us victorious and we will forever walk in that decree forever and ever. In Jesus' Name we pray, Amen!

ABOUT THE AUTHOR

Tony Milton was born on July 30, 1993 in Sarasota, Florida to Tony & Phyllis Milton. He attended Booker High School graduating in 2011. Tony has been on a journey of ministry and purpose, moving into business and the marketplace. His desire is to raise the bar in accomplishments and achievements for young Black men across the world. Tony Milton is the founder and CEO of Milton Bernard Enterprises, LLC which encompasses many different endeavors ranging from books to fashion and all the way to public speaking both in and out of the pulpit. Tony is starting something very new, a new era of young, affluent, godly Black men. Tony Milton is making a point to push the culture forward by challenging all limits and boundaries. Be sure to keep your eyes on all that Tony has in store for the near future.

www.ingramcontent.com/pod-product-compliance
Lightning Source LLC
Chambersburg PA
CBHW071126030426
42336CB00013BA/2214